THE MEDICINE PERSON'S GUIDE TO HERBALISM

Healing with Plant Medicines, Stones, Animal Spirits, and Ceremony

Katie Lynn Sanders, *Bird Woman*

Text Copyright © 2019 Katie Lynn Sanders
All Rights Reserved

Titles by Katie Lynn Sanders

Farmgirl School;
Homesteading 101

From Mama's Kitchen with Love;
New and Old Recipes From our Family

Featherheart Finds Medicine

Homesteader's Pharmacy;
The Complete Guide to Creating Your Own Herbal Pharmacy

The Herbalist Will See You Now;
Your Complete Training Guide to Becoming and Working as an Herbalist

Cherokee Home

The Making of a Medicine Woman;
The Memoirs of Bird Woman

All titles available at AuthorKatieSanders.com

Dedication

To the next generations of Medicine People and my great loves:

My children,

Andrew (*Great Wolf*), Shyanne (*Little Deer*), Emily (*Rabbit*)

And my granddaughters,

Maryjane (*Featherheart*) and Ayla (*Little Eagle*)

Also, to my husband, Doug (*Coyote*), who helps make these books
come to life.

The Medicine Person's Guide to Herbalism

Contents

The Medicine Person's Guide to Herbalism

The Medicine Person's Guide to Herbalism

My Friends,

For the past hundreds of thousands of years, on every continent, there have been medicine people; shamans and wise women, holy people and healers. In their medicine pouches were (are) stones, and magical things of nature, and plants. Plants are the original medicine. The most potent and synergistic of all healers. They can heal on spiritual, emotional, and physical levels. They can carefully heal a broken heart or help someone recover from a heart attack. They can clear negative spirits and they can bring clarity and slow Dementia. They can increase nutrient uptake and mend bones, help with childbirth and stop hemorrhaging. They can bless, they can heal, and they are everywhere one looks.

There are many people who use aloe to heal burns. There are many who can make a lovely tea. Then there are those that are called to be healers. They speak to plants in pleasant tones as they walk by them and the plants respond. They whisper sweetly as if speaking to a child or animal. They hear in their minds what a person needs, what an animal is ailing from, and they use that to create medicine from herbs. Perhaps they are visited by animal spirits and find stones with particular healing properties and they use those as well. Perhaps they need to treat a spiritual ailment or trauma, or perhaps it is simply a cold or bad infection; either way, the medicine person has the sight, the listening skills, and the innate wisdom to create the medicine.

Herbalism is largely intuitive. One can follow recipes and learn the herb's names, identification, and Latin or Native names. One can measure and memorize, but what is most important is to get a good sense of the plants. The practicing medicine person will find that a pinch of this may be needed in one case, but four tablespoons is necessary in another.

I had a student ask me if there was anything that she could use to help her old dog pass peacefully. Alas, I told her, herbs only heal and bless, they do not cause harm. There are no plants that will peacefully cause death. There are poisonous plants out there and it is wise to know them so to avoid them, but almost always, a plant is healing. Do not fear the plants. If you can speak to them and you understand what I am writing, then as long as you know the properties of say, echinacea or elderberries, then you needn't fear. As always, if you feel the person or animal would benefit from modern medical help, do not hesitate to recommend that. After all, we are only vessels of healing and sometimes there is a better way than what we can offer.

In this book I will give you many recipes to help heal common ailments and chronic diseases. Feel free to change them as you intuitively grasp each plant. I encourage you to grow your own plants and wildcraft respectfully. The large corporations and the increased interest in herbalism is causing plants to become endangered and they are vanishing. It is part of our calling as herbalists to grow as much as we can and to educate on the properties of plants while protecting their habitats.

I am excited to bring this book to you. In my last book, *The Homesteader's Pharmacy*, I only included recipes to work with physiological ailments and instructions on to make medicine. In this book, along with many new recipes for physical health, I have included spiritual and emotional uses of plants and recipes. We are not just physical bodies and we are not just spiritual beings, so the medicines must treat every aspect of our being. Sometimes increasing greens will heal an ailment, but sometimes giving up a toxic job will have a more positive effect.

Above all on your journey, always lead with the heart. Always approach from a place of compassion. The plants will never steer you wrong.

Best wishes on your healing journey,

Katie (Bird Woman)

We are medicine women, medicine men, healers, shamans, witches, earth keepers, holy people, guides, herbalists.

A Note About Chakras

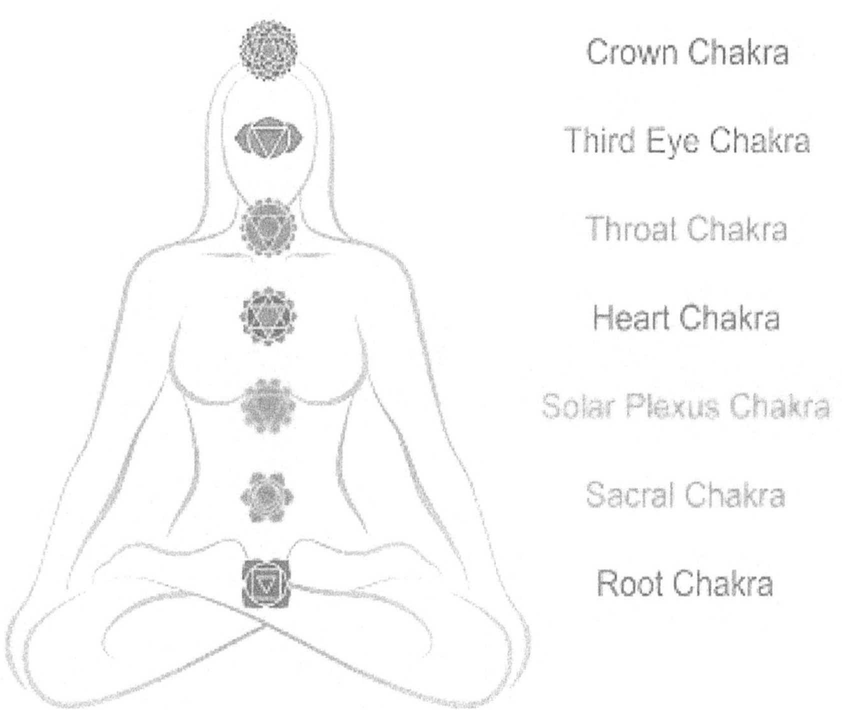

Chakras are also called *Gates* in Cherokee and are known in every culture under different names, but the concept is the same. Our physical bodies are made up of seven energy centers which collect information while we are here and are "loaded" up into the universe upon our death through an 8th chakra, which is believed to be our soul. Lessons that we need to learn, that we have learned, and insight into our ultimate self and physical self are all contained and balanced within the chakras. They are color coded and the ailments that affect the physical body in the area of a specific chakra will be treated the same, whether it is physical or spiritual. This helps the practicing medicine person have further insight into what the client does not say. Almost always, a physical ailment will point to a spiritual unrest, stress, or trauma. Whereas a spiritual ailment can warn of a physical ailment present or approaching.

   The Medicine Person's Guide to Herbalism

1. The Mind

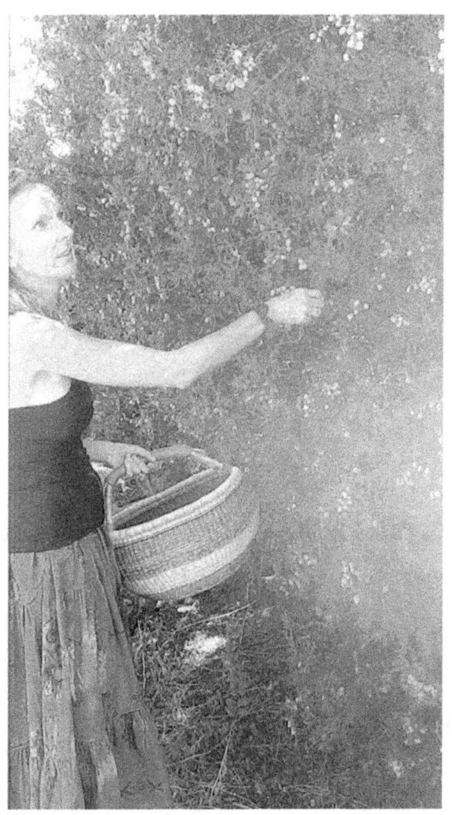

The mind is made up of the brain and the pineal gland (crown chakra and connection to the Divine). Ailments of the brain can be caused from toxins, such as mercury or other metals, stress, and a missing sense of purpose. All these things are remedied by the same herbs in different blends and ratios.

When we are talking about the pineal gland (7th Chakra), we are addressing prayers, connection, purpose, and clarity. The super stars in the plant world for the brain are the very same that medicine people use for prayer and ceremony. The pineal gland governs the thyroid and hormones. If there is spiritual unrest or confusion, one will find the thyroid to be disturbed and stress that needs to be remedied. Physiologically, brain specific herbs are used to help with clarity, focus, energy (thyroid), and to slow diseases, such as Dementia, Cancer, and Alzheimer's. The plant healer will find that someone that has a physiological brain issue (like Dementia or lack of clarity) will be feeling a lack of purpose or spiritual practice. Therefore, someone with a listless sense of purpose may experience lack of clarity and be prone to forgetfulness.

I worked with a Hopi healer as he was preparing a presentation for the medical community on how indigenous people heal Alzheimer's. I was honored that he asked to video tape me speaking as a medicine woman about the herbs that I would use. I would use rosemary for memory. I would add to that sage for wisdom. I would use burdock to ground the person back into their body, as burdock has a very long tap root. This is the spiritual recipe. However, if we look at it scientifically, the rosemary and the sage both have volatile oils which open brain receptors and create alertness, and the burdock cleanses and detoxifies the brain.

As traditional healers, many of us have noted that diseases of the brain, such as Alzheimer's, are simply a way for the body to protect itself from trauma. When an elder loses a spouse, friends, children; if they have memories of war or violence, sometimes it just becomes too much, and their spirit begins to detach from their body. Therefore, we try to mend the body and spirit together in order to be successful. The plants do this for us by intuitively treating both.

Plants that have volatile oils will create alertness and cleanse the brain.

Sage- also used for elders to help remember, symbolic of wisdom, balances estrogen levels, and increases immunity.

Rosemary- also used to increase memory and to recall events and boosts immunity.

Herbs that increase blood flow are important to increase oxygen to the brain.

Gingko- anti-coagulant, increases blood flow to the brain.

Ginger, Turmeric, and other spices- increases blood flow to the brain and lower inflammation.

Herbs that boost immunity and act as adaptogens (increasing the health of the entire body and helping to stabilize the adrenal system) are imperative as they help increase immunity and heal the thyroid while acting to ground because of the tap roots.

Ginseng- repairs adrenals, increases immunity, increases vitality (very endangered)

Ashwagandha- Also very good for the nervous system and for instances of depression. Repairs the adrenals. This herb is special and a bit magical because it helps you "know" the answer. The Divine speaks through this herb.

Dock (burdock, yellow dock, curly dock)- cleansing, grounding, anti-cancer.

Other cleansing herbs that also increase essential nutrients to the brain are green.

Dandelion, Stinging Nettles, Dock leaves, and Purslane (highest form of Omega 3 available).

The herbs and foods for the brain are color coded and are typically brown and green, such as *mushrooms* and *walnuts.* All nuts and seeds and whole grains are specific to brain because they are full of bio-available zinc and other essential vitamins and minerals. *Coffee* is another fabulous herb for the brain! It increases cognitive abilities, memory, focus, increases blood flow to the brain, and is analgesic (pain relieving). Coffee is healthy!

When blending medicines, simply choose one of each category based on what they do.

     The Medicine Person's Guide to Herbalism

Brain Tonic

2 parts each:

Sage

Rosemary

Gingko

Ginseng

Brain Cancer

2 parts each:

Reishi Mushroom

Shitake Mushroom

Chaga Mushroom

Cat's Claw (an herb from Peru)

Alzheimer's Blend

2 parts each:

Foti

Gingko

Gotu Kola

Rosemary

Sage

Borage (anti-depressant)

To Receive Answers and Clarity

Equal parts:

Ashwagandha

Sage

Rosemary

Prepare as an extract or tea and take before meditating on a question.

Other Healing

Animal spirits for healing the mind are owls (wisdom), hawks (focus), and eagles (connection to Spirit), as well as fox (for making quick decisions and observation).

Stones for healing the mind are Amethyst (purple/7th chakra/connection to Spirit), Spirit Quartz, and Purple Fluorite.

Ceremony for healing trauma, for remembering and releasing, and for renewed connection to Spirit may be done with feathers, sage and cedar smoke, and prayers while "cleansing" the top of the head.

  The Medicine Person's Guide to Herbalism

2. The Eyes

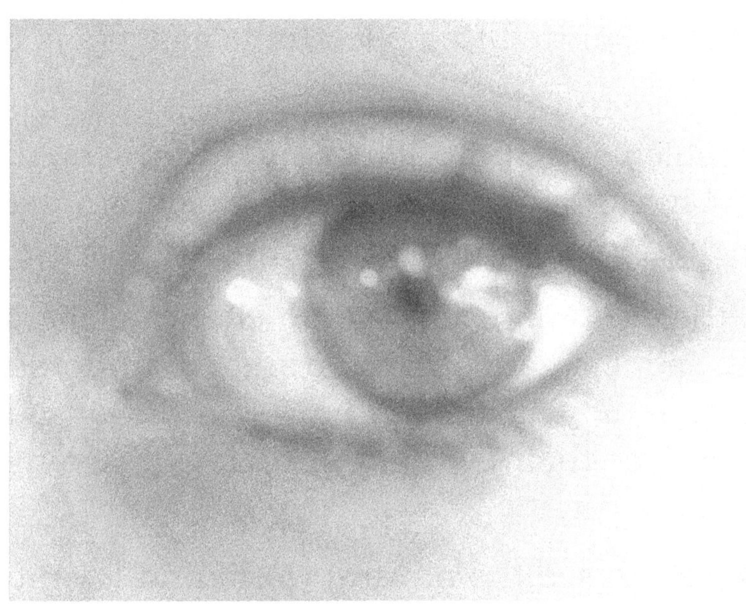

The eyes are fascinating. There are many causes of eye problems. The newest issue facing us today is cell phone and constant computer use. Eye strain is a leading cause of eye sight loss. The lights being emitted from electronic gadgets is certainly causing issues.

Other eye problems include Glaucoma, Cataracts, dry eyes, inflammation, and infection. These can be caused from age, diet, habits, environmental factors, blood pressure, and stress.

Spiritually, the eyes represent the 6th chakra of sight. In the center of the forehead is a gate of all-knowing, of understanding, of "seeing" truths and old wisdoms. I have heard that in some cases psychics that lose their eyesight in turn gain stronger intuition to make up for it.

I love being able to see the natural world and I want to keep my eyes strong.

The Medicine Person's Guide to Herbalism

Eyebright- a quirky plant that resembles an eyeball is my favorite herb for healing eyes. In the middle ages, eyebright was known to "bring people out of blindness." In my experiences, I have found that eyebright (along with its helper herbs) reverse cataracts and glaucoma and help to restore eyesight. Used with cancer herbs, it helps heal cancer of the eye in horses.

Bilberry- this beautiful purple berry is amazing at restoring eyesight.

Yucca- this wonderful western plant is anti-inflammatory. It helps to relieve pressure in the eyes. Yucca contains *saponin,* which is soap. It helps to cleanse the eyes.

Rose Hips- one of the highest forms of Vitamin C and a very good anti-inflammatory.

Elm- the inner bark of all elms (Slippery, Chinese, Siberian) is a soft, *demulcent* medicine that helps sooth irritated membranes.

Mullein- mullein leaf is a wonderful "slippery" herb. The demulcent herbs become gelatinous in their medicinal transport and help to wash out infection and sooth irritated nerves.

Barberry or Oregon Grape Root- I always used *Goldenseal*, but it is becoming very endangered. These three plants contain *berberine*, which is one of the strongest antibiotics available. The yellow color of the root tells of its properties.

Turmeric, Ginger, Gingko, or just barely a pinch of Red Chili Pepper (note- this medicine is *not* going in the eye!)- a good circulatory herb will help the eye medicines work faster. I like to include a circulatory herb in all my medicines to help increase blood flow.

The foods for eyes are yellow. The antioxidant in yellow foods is called Lutein. Orange foods contain beta-carotene, which converts Vitamin A. These fruits and vegetables help to restore health to the eye. Think yellow peppers, corn, egg yolks, yellow squash, yellow carrots, along with orange vegetables and fruits.

Eye Tonic

(Taken by mouth. Not for use in the eye!)

2 parts each:

Eyebright

Bilberry

1 part each:

Yucca

Mullein

Oregon Grape Root

A small piece:

Turmeric or Ginger

This blend is effective to help treat any eye issue.

Eye Healer

(Taken by mouth. Not for use in the eye!)

4 parts Eyebright

2 parts Rose Hips

1 part Yarrow

1 part Inner Elm Bark

1 small piece of Turmeric

Eye Cancer

(Taken by mouth. Not for use in the eye!)

    2 parts Eyebright

    2 parts Echinacea

    2 parts Reishi Mushroom

    2 parts Oregon Grape Root

Eye Wash

This saline solution works for conjunctivitis (eye infection), pink eye, or dry eyes.

2 Tablespoons of Calendula flowers

2 Tablespoons of Comfrey leaf

½ teaspoon of sea salt

Pour over herbs 1 cup of boiling water. Let sit and cool. Strain and keep in refrigerator. Use a cotton ball to squeeze liquid in eye and to wash outer eye.

Add Echinacea for severe infection.

Add Cat's Claw for cancer in horses.

To Increase Intuition

Equal parts:

Eye bright

Bilberry

½ part of pine needles

Prepare as an extract or tea and take before prayers.

Other Healing

Animal Spirits for the eyes are those that are nocturnal with excellent eye sight, such as Owls (wisdom, clairvoyance), Cats (clairvoyance, magic), as well as Coyotes and Wolves. All the above animals have a strong sense of knowing and can see much better than other animals.

Stones used to heal the eyes are typically blue (the color of the Brow chakra), such as Lapis Lazuli, Sapphire, and Celestite.

Ceremony to heal the eyes and increase intuition might include a nighttime ceremony in darkness and silence. Yellow and blue candles may be lit as prayers.

3. Throat, Sinuses, and Lungs

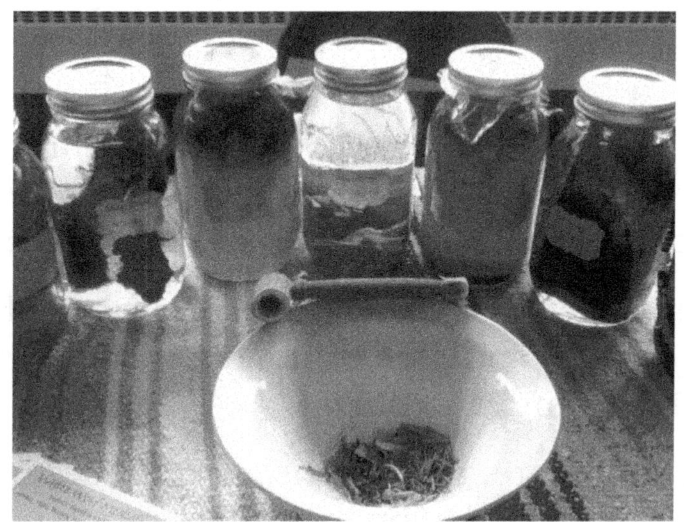

When working with the lungs, sinus cavities, and throat, one is generally addressing immunity. Upper respiratory infections, asthma, and ailments of the lungs, like bronchitis, generally have to do with bacteria, viruses, and common cold symptoms.

The sinuses are moist and perfect breeding grounds for fungus. Pressure headaches, tightness in the face, pressure in the eyes, and cold symptoms often denote a sinus infection.

Lung tissues can be damaged from environmental pollutants causing asthmatic symptoms. Infections or viruses can cause mucous, trouble breathing, and illness.

The throat can be sore, tight, or have an infection from Strep or other viruses. All these ailments can be helped with a basic, strong antibiotic that you can easily brew up. Asthma will have a separate medicine so that it can be used as needed for breathing issues and to strengthen the lungs.

From a spiritual standpoint, these ailments can easily attack someone if they find themselves more stressed than usual. The practicing herbalist will find that stress is the number one exasperator of all ailments. It can cause or worsen acute or chronic ailments.

The fifth chakra is the area that is treated in spiritual and emotional ailments pertaining to the throat. The throat signifies our truth, our voice, and speaking. One might have unexplained tightness in the throat if there is something that they need to say. If a person is not speaking truth (often pertaining to their identity), speaking ill of others, or if they need to follow a different path, the throat will be affected.

The Medicine Person's Guide to Herbalism

Plants

Black Walnut (shells, fruit, or leaves)- this plant is anti-fungal, anti-bacterial, anti-viral, anti-yeast, and is extremely effective in treating sinus infections and yeast infections.

Oregon Grape Root, Barberry, or Goldenseal- our trifecta of berberine-rich plants kill infection- including Staph- in twenty-four hours, in most cases.

Echinacea- this plant (purple coneflower) is a beautiful and well-known plant often associated with colds. But most folks don't fully understand just how powerful this plant is! Anti-viral, anti-cancer, antibiotic, anti-fungal, anti-bacterial, anti-yeast, and immune boosting are just some of the properties of this magnificent plant. I use the leaves and flowers. No use digging up precious roots and destroying the plant.

Mints- any mint will do; chocolate, spearmint, peppermint, orange mint, cat mint, lemon balm, or catnip. The volatile oils in the mint plant opens airways and helps treat common sniffles by drying up the passage ways. It is also a great immune booster and specific to the digestive system.

Mullein flower- the same plant that we use the soft, fuzzy leaves for demulcent uses has medicine atop its stalk! The little yellow flowers will come back each day after harvesting. The humble looking flowers are anti-viral, restore the health of lung tissues, and can help suppress auto-immune issues.

The Medicine Person's Guide to Herbalism

Ephedra and Mormon Tea- essentially the same family, just different continents. They have the same properties. I grow both. They open airways in seconds. They are not commonly available because the FDA doesn't recommend their use (it is not illegal, however) because of the effects of Ephedrine. Once you take a perfectly effective plant into the lab to separate its DNA and constituents to create a patentable lookalike, that is when there becomes problems. It is essentially not the same as the plant, but a chemical version which will always have side effects.

Valerian and Lobelia- these two plants are calmatives. Ephedra and Mormon tea are stimulants. Many times, in herbalism, we use a stimulant and a calmative. This may seem counterproductive, but they work synergistically together to achieve health. In the case of lung health, the stimulant opens airways and forces breath while the calmative sooths and quiets the lungs so that the air can come through. Calmatives will also quiet coughs and help the ailing person relax.

Thyme- this plant contains volatile oils and is immunity boosting. It is specific to lung health (Plants prefer certain systems of the body. Rosemary and sage have volatile oils as well, but they prefer to work with the brain.) and opens airways by increasing breath intake. (Just smell a volatile oil plant like mint, thyme, or eucalyptus to see how it helps one breathe deeper.) Thyme also acts as a circulatory herb by increasing blood flow.

Bear Root (Osha)- Bear root is one of my very favorites. My Hopi friend and teacher taught me about bear root. It is found above

7000 feet above sea level. Taos is a popular place for Natives to gather it. It is a very strong herb. It is an anti-biotic and specific to the throat and the throat chakra. The bears dig it up in the winter time for immunity. It has a very strong, earthy smell and is a limited plant since it cannot readily be cultivated. Bear root is symbolic of the bear and the bear is the animal of herbalists and healers, the keeper of roots. I always keep bear root in my medicine bag for protection. One can burn it as smudge to protect someone or to help heal spiritually. Bear root tea will help one have the bravery to speak their truth and become who they are supposed be.

Foods for the sinuses, lungs, and throat are all immune boosting. Try less meat and more leafy green vegetable and beans. Lungs especially benefit from nightshades, like eggplants and tomatoes. Cinnamon, nutmeg, cardamom, and citruses are very good for the throat.

The Medicine Person's Guide to Herbalism

Strong Antibiotic

2 parts each:

Goldenseal

Oregon Grape Root

Bear Root

Lemon Balm

Sinus Medicine

2 parts each:

Black Walnut

Echinacea

Oregon Grape Root

Mint

Asthma

3 parts Mullein flower and leaf

2 parts Stinging Nettles

1 part each:

Ephedra or Mormon Tea

Lobelia (warning: the other name for this plant is *pokeweed*, don't use too much!)

½ part each:

Ginger

Thyme

Cold/Flu

3 parts Elder berry

2 parts Echinacea

2 parts Mint

1 part Mullein flower

Throat Spray

2 parts each:

Bear root

Echinacea

Mint

Cinnamon

Prepare as an extract then cut 50% with water and put in spray bottle.

For Courage to Become One's True Self

Equal parts

Bear Root

Cinnamon

Mint

Prepare as extract, tea, or spray for throat or self and take during meditations.

The Medicine Person's Guide to Herbalism

Other Healing

Animal Spirits for throat are song birds, blue jays, and bear.

Stones for the throat chakra are turquoise or blue. Try turquoise (the healer's stone), Aquamarine, and Kyanite.

Ceremony for the throat and speaking one's truth and for bravery may include feathers, cedar, tobacco and bear root as smudge, singing, drumming, and turquoise colored candles.

4. Heart and Nervous System

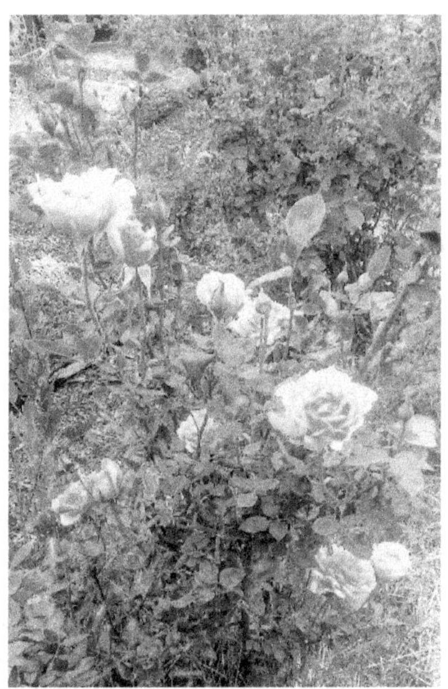

Out of the thousands of people I have helped over the years, I do believe that ailments of the nervous system and the heart have been the most prevalent of cases. And nearly always, they coincide with the spiritual aspect of these systems. Heartbreak, trauma, and stress cause more heart attacks and chronic pain issues than any other, in my experience.

The nervous system governs sleep, stress, and pain. If a person is experiencing problems with one, they are likely experiencing problems with the others. The nervous system governs the digestive system so stomach problems often occur when stress is a problem. The nervous system is governed by the heart and mind.

I read a journal from the Civil War that spoke of women dying of broken hearts after their men were killed in battle. For centuries medicine people have known that heartache causes heart attacks. They are directly related. I believe that is why women die of heart attacks more than any other ailment. Women tend to take on the burdens of the world and the stresses of others.

Scientifically speaking, the medical community is realizing that the outer muscle of the heart loosens during heartbreak and stress. The herbs that we use for the heart strengthen that muscle and increase oxygen. Under stress, we tend to hold our breath. The circulatory system goes under attack.

I have witnessed incidences of severe, long term chronic pain occurring after a fight with a loved one. I have seen strokes and heart attacks occur after the loss of a spouse. I have seen stress cause insomnia, anger, and numbness, and even cancer. This is a very important system to understand. The healing process goes much deeper than what is on the surface or what a client may initially divulge.

This system also includes the veins; thrombosis, varicose veins, blood clotting issues, and blood flow.

Hawthorn- my ultimate favorite tree. It is the most beautiful, unassuming tree that one might stumble upon in the woods. At first, one sees the berries and wonders what type of tree it might be. The leaves look like currants. The tree stands about ten feet high. If one looks closely, the thorns appear. Long, sharp, sometimes two inches in length, thorns set crisply between twigs and branches. These berries and leaves literally heal broken hearts. Hawthorn also strengthens the muscles of the heart and the veins.

Rose- the plant that symbolizes love. It also signifies love for oneself. It helps one forgive and move forward. To proceed with compassion and love. Physiologically, rose's properties sooth the nervous system and clear the skin. It is uplifting and a mild anti-depressant.

St. John's Wort- one of my very favorites. This plant is so powerful that its constituents have been isolated and changed chemically to become popular pharmaceuticals like Prozac, Gabapentin, Wellbutrin, Cymbalta, and many other anti-depressants and chronic pain relievers. The pharmaceuticals are lab created so therefore will have harsh side effects that one would not experience with the straight plant medicine. St. John's Wort is the *only* plant that will interact with pharmaceutical anti-depressants and chronic pain relievers made from its derivatives. If it is an MAOI (monoamine oxidase inhibitor), then St. John's Wort will wash it out of the system leaving the client with withdrawals. If a person is off their anti-depressants for 24 hours, they can safely go on St. John's Wort blends. If someone is on MAOI pharmaceuticals, give them medicines that do not contain St. John's Wort.

Borage- the strongest anti-depressant after St. John's Wort. This lovely plant has spiky leaves and starburst blue flowers. Its properties are very strong, but as with all plants, you cannot overdose on it. It is a lovely, uplifting, nerve strengthening and healing plant.

California Poppy- this yellow buttercup-looking flower and its leaves are in the poppy family, but do not contain opiates. They can, however, help someone get off opiates. The effects of California Poppy can be as strong as morphine, but without side effects, making it a very good plant to have in one's apothecary.

Valerian- valerian out of a lab becomes Valium. It is an excellent calmative and pain reliever. It steadies the nerves, helps one sleep well, and helps heal nerve damage. Valerian root can be used in ceremony to help speak to spirits. It is quite strong, and I do prefer to use the leaves and flowers in my extracts.

Skullcap- this is the very best herb to stop and control seizures. It is a great calmative and nerve healer.

Chamomile, Lavender, Lemon Verbena, Catnip, Lemon balm, and Jasmine- plants such as these are considered "supporting actors" in my medicines. Valerian, St. John's Wort, and California Poppies are rather strong and work better blended with similar, but more soothing herbs. I generally use 2 parts strong herb to 1

   The Medicine Person's Guide to Herbalism

part supporting. All of these are very good for children and animals.

Yarrow, Witch hazel, Butcher's Broom, Horse Chestnut, and Oak- these are all fabulous vein healers and they consistently control blood flow through the veins. Herbs balance, there cannot be too much or too little, for they will work themselves out! So, these work as blood thinners or thickeners depending on what is needed. They are effective at healing thrombosis, inner blood clots, varicose veins, spider veins, and circulatory issues.

Foods that heal the heart are red/pink and green. The very same colors as the heart chakra. Anthocyanins can be found in wine, grapes, tomatoes (they have four chambers, just like the heart), beets, berries, and red peppers. Add in greens like kale, spinach, and allicins (white plants), such as garlic and onion.

Foods that heal the nervous system all have a soothing quality, such as oils like olive, coconut, and sunflower, nuts and seeds, and whole grains.

Nerve Pain/Repair

2 parts each:

Valerian

St. John's Wort

Skullcap

California Poppy

1 part Chamomile

Heart

3 parts each:

Hawthorn berries and/or leaves

Mistletoe leaf (blood pressure)

1 part each:

Yarrow

Motherwort

A small piece of ginger

Sleep Well

2 parts each:

Valerian

Skullcap

California Poppy

1 part each:

Chamomile

Hops

Stress Free

> 3 parts each:
> St. John's Wort
> Borage
> 1 part each:
> Lemon Balm
> Roses

Calm Spirit

> 2 parts each:
> Hawthorn
> Borage
> Catnip
> Lemon Balm
> Roses

Anti-Seizure

> 2 parts each:
> Valerian
> Skullcap
> Cat's Claw (suppresses auto-immune response and "misfiring" of the brain)
> California Poppy

Varicose Vein

2 parts each:

Witch hazel

Oak leaves

Yarrow

Hawthorn

Use extract as topical liniment.

To Open One's Heart

Equal parts:

Hawthorn

Rose

Maple

Take as a tea or extract daily.

Other Healing

Animal spirits for heart are deer (gentleness of spirit), dog (loyalty and friendship), and hummingbird (love).

Stones that can be used to heal the heart and heartbreak are pink, such as pink Quartz, pink Opal, and Rhodonite. Blood stone is a powerful healer.

Ceremony for healing heart break will often include delicious teas of heart specific herbs and a healing ceremony with stones and clearing with cedar, sweetgrass, tobacco, and sage.

5. Solar Plexus and Organs

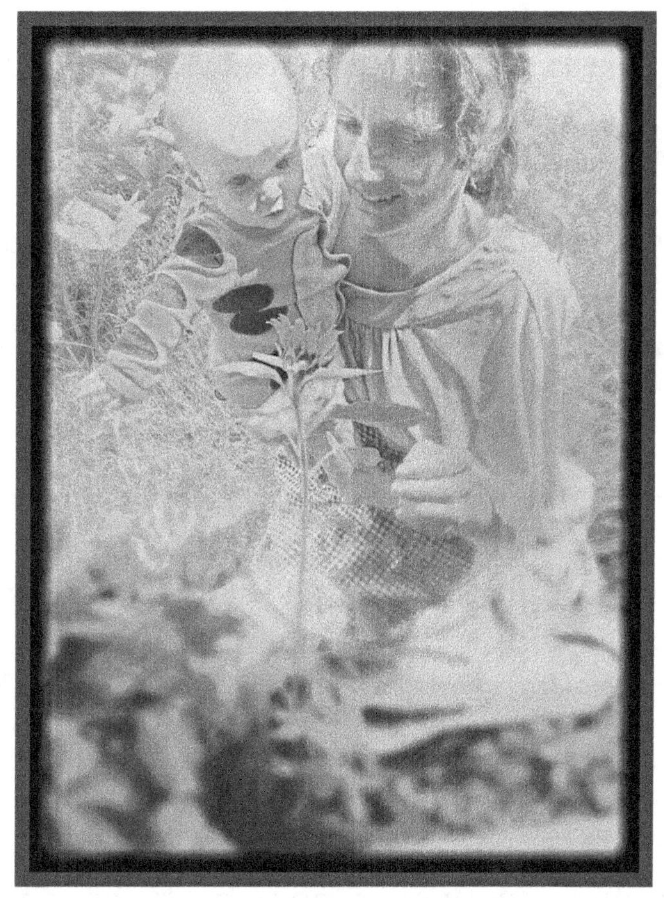

The Medicine Person's Guide to Herbalism

I had an extremely strong, annoying sensation in my gut. It felt like someone was kicking me in the diaphragm. It made me angry and listless. I was so distracted by it that I nearly got in a car accident with my three small children in the backseat. I prayed that I could find an answer to what this pressing feeling was.

A short time later I was walking through a book store with my family and saw a colorful book displayed on an endcap. It showed the figure of a body and seven energy circles in vibrant colors. There was a bright yellow globe on the figure that corresponded directly to where the problem was on me. I bought the book.

The kicked-in-the-gut feeling was not a physical ailment. It felt like a bit of anxiety, but it really was not something that I could not point out as a physical injury. My solar plexus, I learned, was the place within that holds one's power. A place where all the talents, gifts, and paths in the world are held.

I had long "shut off" my psychic abilities. It scared me to sense spirits and I was terrified of being possessed. My mother was certain my gifts were not of God. I used to dream about the news in detail, watching every gory moment, before the news even aired. I "knew" and "saw" way too much for me to be able to deal with. I was a young mother and wife and I had no idea what to do with these powers. So, I shut them off and they were limited to knowing when the phone was about to ring.

They were trying to come forth in the most forceful way. They would not be quieted any longer. It was soon after that incident that I learned about herbs as healing medicines and realized that my psychic abilities led me to be able to "see" ailments, injuries, and diseases in others and helped me know what herbs to put together for them.

                                   The Medicine Person's Guide to Herbalism

A few years after that, various medicine people stepped forward to teach me ceremonial healing and spiritual ways of healing. I take breaks from my work to restore but as long as I don't completely shut it off, my solar plexus doesn't cause trouble.

I combined the solar plexus with treating organs in this chapter because the solar plexus is a place of power and when folks aren't pursuing their divine path, stuff falls apart. Anger is held in the liver. Grief and feeling like a victim are held in the spleen and pancreas. The organs work constantly to help clear blood and distribute nutrients, produce hormones, and keep the body running. Besides emotions, the biggest cause of organ failure is diet. Our world is filled with made-made chemicals, metals, and poisons that are infiltrating our bodies from everywhere. From the air we breathe to the food and water we consume, we are being inundated with poisonous materials. Cleansing is incredibly important. Not harsh laxatives, but easy, nutrient-rich plants that can quickly restore health to the organs.

In order to live our absolute truth, our divine purpose, and our best life, we must take care of our bodies as well as our gifts.

The Medicine Person's Guide to Herbalism

Calendula- this herb is cleansing, anti-cancer, anti-viral, and skin clearing. Its spiritual properties are specific to the solar plexus. Plants that look like the sun represent the chakra where our power and gifts are held.

Sunflower- specific to the skin, cleansing, and is soothing to the system. It is used to boost immunity and is high in Vitamin E. The sunflower follows the sun, its head is a vibrant yellow or orange and represents the solar plexus. The solar plexus is the place of fun, sun, and child-like wonder. It is the place that we can be ourselves.

Dandelion- specific to the liver and gallbladder. Mild laxative and diuretic. Extremely healing. Washes out cancer cells.

Stinging Nettles- controls allergies, works as an anti-histamine, clears sinuses, and cleanses the blood. Increases breast milk and is very nutrient rich. Cleanses organs.

Docks- curly, yellow, and burdock are all amazing sources of minerals and vitamins. They cleanse the lymphatic system completely, ushering out dead and cancerous cells. The leaves flush the organs.

Purslane- highest form of Omega 3's, common garden weed, demulcent, specific to brain and pancreas. Helps with insulin production.

Prickly Pear- an extremely cleansing and healing plant. The inner gel stabilizes the pancreas and can help reverse Diabetes.

Foods that heal the organs are all dark and leafy green; kale, spinach, collards, and mustards. Ethnic spices are all very good at restoring health to the organs, specifically the pancreas. Cinnamon, cardamom, nutmeg, red chili, and pepper are all great mixed into extracts, teas, and coffee. Citrus peels can be dried and added to help stimulate metabolism and control Diabetes. Green tea is an antioxidant rich and healing drink. Orange is specific to the lymphatic system and heals all cancers. Try carrots, orange peppers, winter squashes, and oranges.

Foods that help the solar plexus would be citruses and brightly colored fruits and flowers. Anti-anxiety/anti-depressant herbs are wonderful for this system as well.

Allergy

4 parts each:

Stinging Nettles

Elder Flower

Anti-Cancer

2 parts each:

Agrimony

Cat's Claw

Mistletoe Leaves

Dandelion

Detox

2 parts each:

Bear grass (the fronds from the yucca plant)

Dandelion

Stinging Nettles

Burdock

Diabetes

1 part each:

Dandelion

Mullein Leaf

Ginseng

Cinnamon

Bay

Gingko

Ginger

Parsley

Prickly Pear or Aloe frond

Digestive

1 part each:

Mint

Lemon Balm

Chamomile

Ginger

Mullein Leaf

Fennel

Anise

Turmeric

Kidney/Bladder

2 parts each:

Frozen or fresh Cranberries

Corn silk

Echinacea

Juniper Berries

Skin Clear

2 parts each:

Calendula

Agrimony

Red Clover

Dandelion

Weak Bladder

2 parts each:

Agrimony

Ephedra

Sumac

Horsetail

   The Medicine Person's Guide to Herbalism

Weight Loss

2 parts each:

Dried Orange Peel

Dandelion

1 part each:

Cinnamon

Ginger

Turmeric

Ginseng

Gingko

To Accept Gifts, Talents, Powers to Heal

Equal parts:

Calendula

Sunflowers

Borage

Make into extract or tea and take during meditation.

Animal spirits to help heal the solar plexus and come into one's own power and accept divine gifts and guidance are large cats (courage, strength), specifically tigers, usually white, house cats (magic), wolf (bettering those around you, loyalty, powerful), and one's own spirit animal.

Stones for the 3rd chakra are yellow, such as amber or topaz. Also, smoky quartz used as protection as you accept your gifts.

Ceremony- a rite of passage may be of use, a gathering of like-minded holy people to surround the person with love and protection. Smudging with flowers and cedar, bells, and singing and dancing can all help a person come into their own power. Calendula teas and sunflowers are called for. Yellow candles would be lovely.

6. Sacral and Hormones

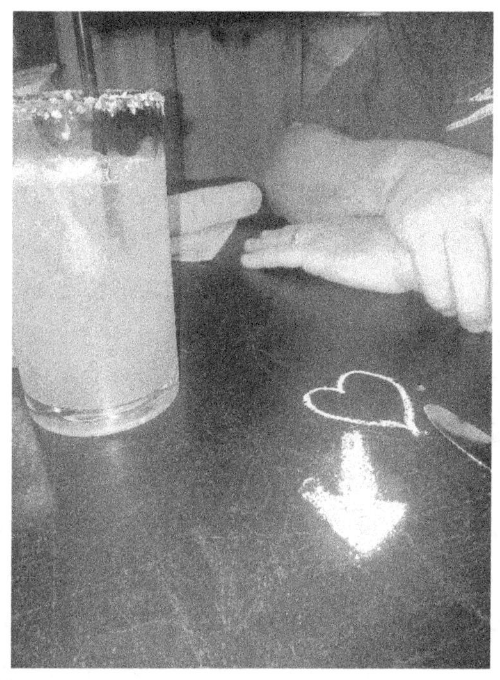

The Medicine Person's Guide to Herbalism

The sacral chakra represents fire and life. Being truly human while we are here. Sometimes as medicine people, we find ourselves locked into our spiritual side- kind of out there in the ether- and it is hard to be grounded.

But being human means that we have the marvelous gifts of sensory. We can taste sweet candies, and salty chips, savory sauces, or delicious wines. We can feel the soft fur of an animal or the sweet arms around us of a hug. We can hear the ocean waves and birds call. We can smell the damp earth after the rain or the new growth in the forest. We can see the sunset and the layers of stars and a deer with her fawn. We feel empathy, joy, freedom, sadness, guilt, grief, anger, then happiness again in our circle of lessons and experiences. Being human means that we can (and should) drink the coffee, taste the French food, watch and walk through nature, enjoy sensual pleasures with a partner, and be fully present during this amazing human journey.

If our sacral chakra is off, it can denote a lack of these joys. Perhaps a person has become guarded after sexual trauma, or perhaps being heartbroken after a partner passes, lack of trust, and depression can all cause the 2nd chakra to be blocked, causing not only lack of life force, but also hormone and sexual issues. Note that the pineal chakra was our connection to Spirit, and it too, can cause hormone disruptions. All the systems of the body work together to be balanced and whole so that we can experience our time here as fully as possible, spiritually and physically.

The Medicine Person's Guide to Herbalism

Plants

Black Cohosh- this plant is also called *ganage* in Cherokee, which means, *snake root.* Learning the herb names in different languages helps us to understand their uses. Black Cohosh is often thought of for hot flashes. However, sage is much better for hot flashes. Black cohosh helps to balance estrogen levels. (Remember that plants do not contain hormones; they make the body produce the right amount of hormones.) Black Cohosh is also an excellent muscle relaxer.

Blue Cohosh- Blue Cohosh also balances estrogen levels. A combination of black and blue cohosh can help ready the uterus for childbirth. (As such, one wouldn't use it during pregnancy until it is time to give birth!) Blue cohosh also contains berberine, making it a great medicine to help prevent and treat yeast infections.

Sage- Wise woman-Sage woman, same meaning! Sage (culinary sage, pasture wort (aka: lady sage by the Hopi), and wild sage all can be used) will control hot flashes and balance estrogen levels.

Mugwort- Mugwort is a magical herb that can be used to induce dreams and prophesies when placed under one's pillow. It also balances estrogen levels and is anti-fungal and anti-yeast.

Red Clover- balances all the hormones, but specifically estrogen. It is used in the treatment of breast cancer and is a beautiful detoxifying herb.

Wild Yam- this plant balances progesterone. It controls blood flow and can stop a miscarriage. It is also anti-inflammatory.

Saw Palmetto- this plant balances progesterone as well and is specific to men (though it works for women as well). It is anti-inflammatory and is very good for the prostate.

Motherwort- this herb helps balance all the hormones in the body and helps restore health to the thyroid.

Ginseng- this herb is an adaptogen and helps balance testosterone. It can heal the thyroid completely and is great for vitality, immunity, and energy.

Vanilla- this herb is not only delicious, but it is used to help with sexual performance. It balances testosterone levels.

Damiana- this beautiful herb is used to help with sexual disfunction and to heal the heart as well as increasing arousal. It balances testosterone.

Remember, herbs balance! Both females and males make and use all hormones. The kidneys produce the most hormones. The "fight or flight" syndrome of always being stressed and in a hurry affect the thyroid and adrenals. Choose one herb for each hormone and a balancer to make a hormone medicine.

The Medicine Person's Guide to Herbalism

Foods for the adrenal system and hormone production, as well as for sacral health, are seafood (Iron, Vitamin D), fruits, and chocolate. Greens should be added to the diet to assist in every system.

Recipes

Balanced Hormone

> 1 part each:
>
> Black Cohosh
>
> Wild Yam
>
> Sage
>
> Licorice
>
> Chaste Berry
>
> Motherwort
>
> Red Clover

In the Mood for Love

> 3 parts each:
>
> Vanilla
>
> Damiana
>
> Hawthorn

Prostate

> 2 parts each:
>
> Saw Palmetto
>
> Cranberry
>
> 1 part each:
>
> Corn Silk
>
> Parsley
>
> Ginger
>
> Ginseng

The Medicine Person's Guide to Herbalism

Thyroid

2 parts each:

Black Cohosh

Saw Palmetto

Motherwort

Ginseng

To Increase Sensory

Equal parts:

Red Rose

Vanilla

Strawberry

Make into an extract with honey or into tea and take as needed.

Animal Spirits that can be beneficial for the sacral chakra are rabbit (fertility), wolf (family), and eagle (divine love of fertility and family).

Stones that are orange are used to heal the sacral chakra, such as Carnelian, Halite, and Crocoite.

Ceremony to release sexual traumas and grief over loss (usually of a child) are private. A simple heat proof container of tobacco and roses to pray with as smudge and an orange candle etched with prayers can help release that darkness.

7. Root Chakra and Skeletal System

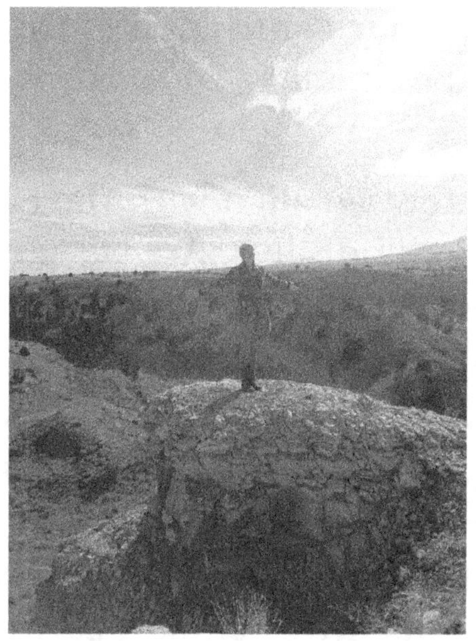

The pineal gland and top of the head (which includes the mind) is connected to the entire universe and star people, then the root at the base of our spine is connected to the earth and of what we are made of. It is our connection to the planet; to earth, to the plants and trees, the animals, the soil. We are the earth and it is us.

The root chakra is how we align with the earth. Are we connected? Are we living mindfully? Are we settled and rooted, or in transition and listless? All these things can play a factor in the health of the 1st chakra.

I combined the skeletal system with the root chakra because our human form is made up of our bones, ligaments, muscles, and tendons, and it all returns to the earth. I buried the ashes of my dear friend, Kat, and upon moving homes, I dug her back up, carefully looking for the bone fragments. I carried with me my grandmother's ashes as well and placed them beneath a stone heart and planted a grape vine. From dust we came and to dust we will return.

Being connected to the natural world around us is every bit as important as being connected to a higher source. We are equal parts body and spirit and our emotions are between those. To be completely well physically and spiritually, we must take care of our bodies and souls.

The natural world helps us so much as Medicine People. From the animal spirits, the plant medicines, the stones, the elements, and seasons all help us in our work. They are directly connected to Spirit and there are no differences between above and below.

To feel rooted, secure, and settled is imperative to creating a calming, happy, fulfilling lifestyle and to be the best healer you can be.

Roots of all sorts- help us spiritually ground and connect with the earth. Burdock, yellow dock, curly dock, ginseng, bear root, and comfrey.

Tree Medicine- is very grounding. The leaves of maple help heal the spirit and ground us to a place. Oak is cleansing and strengthening. Willow is healing. Trees, with their long, old roots help us grow our own.

Willow, Cottonwood, Aspen, Birch- these trees, especially all willows, have analgesic properties. A constituent from willow was the original aspirin. Aspirin is *salicylic acid* whereas Willow contains *salicin.* A big difference; both help sore and swollen muscles and pain, help break fevers, and help the heart, but the willow is the only one without side effects! Analgesic herbs won't heal nerve damage, like nervines do (St. John's Wort, Valerian, et cetera). They are specific to achiness, arthritis, or injury-type pain.

Yucca- I adore this plant and they are prevalent on my western land. The plant is what Native Americans used to make soap to wash themselves and clothes. The saponin content of yucca is great for cleansing wounds. Its anti-inflammatory properties are what draws me to it time and time again.

Cramp Bark- when I was a child growing up in Denver, I knew these bushes as Snowball bush. Large hydrangea-looking flowers

hung heavy on large bushes throughout the city. The inner bark
of this plant is an amazing muscle relaxer.

Dandelion- I use this plant a lot because it is so common. When
healing skeletal issues, especially arthritis ailments (Rheumatoid
Arthritis, Gout, Lupus, Chronic Pain Disorders), cleansing the
tissues is of the utmost importance. The toxins in the tissues is
the very thing the body is attacking!

Cat's Claw or St. John's Wort- both herbs have the amazing ability
to cleanse the blood and tissues while suppressing the
autoimmune response that keeps the body attacking itself.

Comfrey- this is another plant that the FDA unfairly rules unsafe.
The varietal that the agency speaks of is extinct and the pitifully
small study (twelve people) was definitely biased. I have seen
comfrey heal cancer, and I suppose that is not something that big
pharma wants folks to know. Its other amazing use is that it
heals broken bones in two weeks. Everything I mention here, I
have seen in my own work. Animals, children, and many adults,
from butterfly breaks, collar bones, to shattered ankles, all healed
in two weeks or less with comfrey.

Horsetail- this is a fun plant to harvest. It is a reed, usually
hidden amongst high grasses. Once you see one, you find dozens
more! This plant contains silica, making it amazing for repairing
nails, hair, and bones. The plant looks like broken bones pinned
together.

Circulatory Herbs- herbs to increase circulation help get the
medicine through the system faster and help move blood to
decrease pain. Ginger, Turmeric or Cinnamon are good.

　　　　　　　　　　　　　　　The Medicine Person's Guide to Herbalism

Volatile Oils- the hot oils in Cedar, Mint, Eucalyptus, Pine, and Rosemary made into an extract to be used topically nearly instantly stop pain in muscles and tissues and heal the injury very quickly.

Plants that heal the skeletal system are cabbage, organic soybeans, salmon, mushrooms, and dark, leafy greens.

Arthritis

2 parts Willow Bark

1 part each:

Yucca

Rose hips

Cramp Bark

Cat's Claw

Devil's Claw (an anti-inflammatory)

½ part Ginger or Turmeric

Fever Reducer and Migraine Medicine

3 parts each:

Feverfew

Willow Bark

1 part each:

Mint

Catnip

Muscle Healing Liniment

1 part each:

Willow Bark

Oak Leaves

Yucca Root

Cedar or Pine (a six-inch section from a tree branch)

Mint

California Poppy

Comfrey

Make into an extract and apply topically.

Bone Healer

3 parts Comfrey

2 parts each:

Horsetail

St. John's Wort

1 part Arnica

To Feel Grounded and Content

Equal parts:

Burdock

Oak leaves

Wild sage

The Medicine Person's Guide to Herbalism

Prepare as an extract or tea and take during meditation while feeling the base of your spine become a root that burrows deep into the earth. A purple light releases from the top of your head and connects to the powers that be. Feel grounded and filled with gratitude.

Other Healing

Animal spirits for rootedness and connecting with the earth are snake (lives among rocks or in the ground. Keeper of special medicine), bear (roots for medicines), and turtle (spirit animal of earth, the original inhabitant).

Stones for healing the root chakra are red, such as Red Calcite, Red Jasper, and Mookaite. There are earth stones as well that are very healing. If you see one that attracts you, ask it if you may use it.

Ceremony will be in nature with trees and plants around. The wilder the better. A shell with tobacco, cedar, sage, sweet grass, and bear root will help your prayers extend further and help ground. A meditation where one can imagine a light shooting up through the top of their head connecting them to the infinite stars and the universe and one shooting down through the base of the spine firmly into the earth will help balance and ground the spirit.

The Medicine Person's Guide to Herbalism

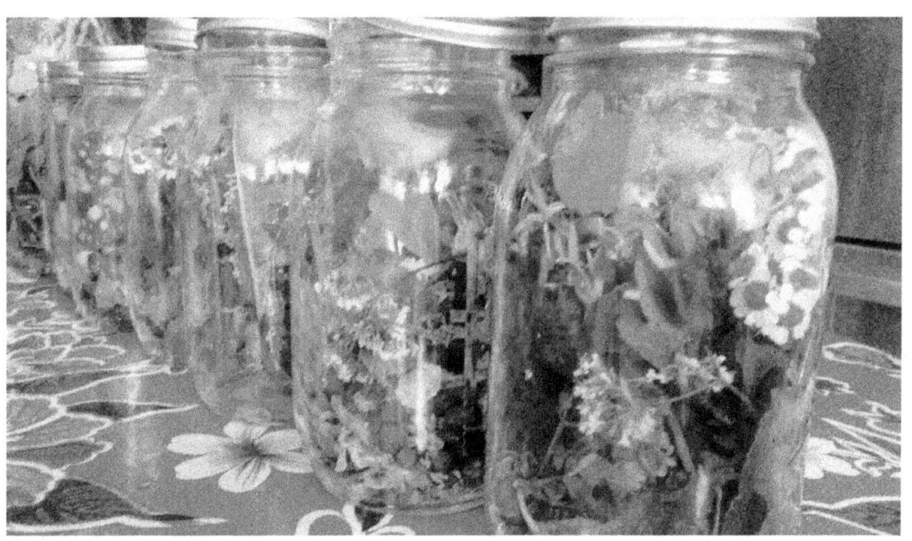

The Medicine Person's Guide to Herbalism

Extracts

Every herbalist develops their own way of creating extracts/tinctures. Extracts are the pure, uncut mother that is made with a ratio of plants and an extracting agent, usually alcohol, sometimes vinegar. The uncut medicine is by far the most effective and strongest, but a little rough to get down!

In a quart sized canning jar:

Add 8 tablespoons of herbs (fresh or dried)

Fill to one inch head space with any 80 proof alcohol like vodka, or rum.

This beautiful potion goes into the sunshine (outdoors if possible, if not, the windowsill is fine) and sits for a few days. Then I put it back on the shelf until the night before the full moon. The full moon changes the frequency of the medicine to match the human body's. Fascinating, isn't it? Don't be alarmed when the herbs begin to move, the color changes, and the lid pops all night. I leave this concoction (clearly marked with a sharpie!) in the moon for a few nights. The medicine is done in four weeks. Do not strain. Just take what you need. This extract is good forever.

The typical dosage of a 100% extract is 2 droppers (1 teaspoon) per day for tonics, 3x a day for acute illness. Or up to 6 droppers 3x a day for severe pain. Halve that for children and halve it even further for animals over 20 pounds. Babies and small animals can use a glycerite.

The Medicine Person's Guide to Herbalism

Gas Reliever

2 Tablespoons each:

Fennel

Anise

Peppermint

Chamomile

Add herbs and rum into a 1 quart canning jar and brew as listed above.

The Medicine Person's Guide to Herbalism

Alcohol, Honey, and Water Tinctures

This is my new way of making medicine for our home use. I love the flavor. At home, I brew these in one gallon drink dispensers so that I have plenty on hand. I simply open the spout and pour half a shot glass full. I take a higher dose because it is cut, but I made more, and it is easy to take.

First, I brew the quart of alcohol. I double the amount of plants to 16 Tablespoons of herbs. I typically make these medicines during the growing season because I love using fresh herbs. I love how beautiful they look while brewing. Just fill the jar (not too tight) with herbs and then pour vodka over the herbs to 1 inch head space and seal. Mark with a sharpie and process like one would do the Extracts.

Pour finished extract into one gallon container (I don't strain it) and add 1 quart of honey and 2 quarts of fresh water. Let this brew another month, stirring occasionally. Eventually the honey does combine with the rest of the medicine. This extract will stay good for many years.

Happy Heart

(an anti-depressant)

> St. John's Wort
>
> Borage
>
> Lemon Balm
>
> Catnip
>
> Roses
>
> Lavender
>
> Hawthorn
>
> I intuitively pick the flowers and leaves and place them into the jar. They may end up being equal parts.

Even Stronger Antibiotic

(lord, this stuff is hard to get down)

> A large root of Oregon Grape
>
> 4 inch piece of Bear Root
>
> 2 Tablespoons of Goldenseal leaf
>
> Echinacea leaves and flowers
>
> Burdock leaves and a 3 inch root
>
> A handful of Juniper berries
>
> Prepare as an extract with vodka in a quart canning jar then follow instructions to make it with honey and water.

The Medicine Person's Guide to Herbalism

Vinegar/ Agave Extract

Vinegar will not extract as well as alcohol, but many folks prefer to abstain from spirits, so vinegar will work. Use dried herbs when you can so the mixture doesn't rot. The agave makes it quite palatable and is low on the glycemic index. It is essentially processed aloe. The herbs change the spirit of the alcohol and other ingredients into medicine.

Use the same technique as making an Extract. Use 8 Tablespoons of herbs. Put in a quart jar and fill jar ¾ of the way full with organic apple cider vinegar. Then top with organic agave.

Let that brew for 3 days in the sun, put on shelf, 3 days in the full moon. Then repeat for another month. The vinegar takes 2 months before it is ready. Then the dosage is twice as much. This is a great way to treat kids. Vinegar extracts are good for two years.

Cold and Flu Remedy

3 Tablespoons of dried Elderberries

2 Tablespoons each:

Dried Echinacea root, flower, or leaves

Dried Mint

½ Tablespoon each:

Feverfew

Valerian

Place herbs in a quart sized canning jar and fill ¾ with apple cider vinegar and ¼ agave. Prepare as an extract.

Teas are an amazing way to make medicine. So long as the herb is fairly tasty, one can blend what is needed and what is on hand to quickly prepare medicine. Add honey to sweeten.

The standard ratio to make tea is 1 teaspoon of dried herbs to 1 cup of boiling water. Using intuition and taste preference, adjust amount of herbs used. This is the standard recipe for leaves and flowers.

For decocting roots and hard shells, simmer in pot of water for 40 minutes. 1 inch of roots per 1 cup of water. Add a bit more to allow for evaporation.

Tea is ceremonial. It is grounding and helps connect us to others.

I use teas when I need to flush a system, such as the cases of parasites, kidney stones, or bacterial infections in the digestive system.

Teas are lovely to give for colds and flus and to settle an upset stomach. Teas can be made like iced tea and carried throughout the day. Spiritual teas are very powerful and lovely to consume.

Heartbreak Tea

2 parts each:

Hawthorn berries

Rose petals

Lemon Balm

1 part each:

Lavender

Yarrow

½ part Ginger

Brew strong and pour into quart jars with ice to sip during the day. 2 quarts and ceremony tend to heal a broken heart from neglect, rejection, or disappointment.

Glycerite

Glycerin is kind of a product of unknown history, but essentially it is the by-product of the vegetable industry. Either way, it is the best transport for baby and small animal medicine.

Use 2 parts herbs to 3 parts glycerin. Use your judgement, if it is too thick, add more glycerin, not enough herbs, add more.

Very slowly, heat over medium-low heat in a saucepan, swirling often, until the glycerin is colored and looks like the consistency of hot honey, about 25 minutes. When you begin to smell the herbs, it is finished. Let cool for a few moments then slowly add a dash of apple cider vinegar and immediately strain into a canning jar. Concoction will be hot!

The vinegar is to make the glycerin less thick so that one can use a dropper bottle to dispense. This medicine is good for about two years.

The dosage is 1 dropper, 2 if it is an acute situation.

Puppy Anxiety and Baby Teething Relief

2 parts Valerian

2 parts Chamomile

Pour three times as much glycerin over herbs and slowly heat for about 25 minutes. Pour in a splash of apple cider vinegar and strain into clean jar. Apply to sore teeth, or give 1 dropper to dogs, cats, and babies who refuse to sleep.

Infused Honey

Making infused honey is quick and easy. It is excellent to put in tea (using a strainer) and is great way to get kids to take their medicine.

Place 1 Tablespoon of dried herbs in a 4 ounce canning jar and top with honey, leaving ½ inch headspace. Replace lid and put in sauce pan of boiling water covering. Boil for 5 minutes.

You can make several different kinds of infused honey this way and prepare them all at the same time. Infused honey never goes bad so long as you use dried herbs.

Allergy Honey

(honey has a small medicinal effect on seasonal allergies, but when added to anti-allergy herbs, the medicine is great.)

2 teaspoons of dried Stinging Nettles

1 teaspoon of dried Dandelion

Top with local honey and prepare as above.

Infused Oil

Infused oil can be used to treat ear infections (garlic and willow oil) or turned into salves and creams or used as is. Always use dried herbs to prevent mold.

In a pint-sized canning jar, add 4 Tablespoons of dried herbs and top with oil, leaving ½ inch head space. Put lid loosely on and mark with a sharpie what it is. Place in sunny window for 2 weeks. After a few days you can replace lid tighter and shake a few times a day.

Oil keeps for at least a year. Try sunflower, safflower, or olive oil. Any additions to the oils, like aloe or coconut oil, will cause the concoction to go rancid in a month.

Nerve Pain and Bruising Oil

3 Tablespoons of St. John's Wort

1 Tablespoon of Arnica

One could also make this into a salve by double boiling ½ ounce of beeswax with 1 cup of infused oil.

Vapor Oil

(Use this to open airways by rubbing on chest)

1 Tablespoon each:

Cedar (fresh)

Peppermint

Eucalyptus

Rosemary

I would never recommend someone to take essential oils internally. They are very strong. Essential oils have some topical healing abilities when properly cut but their real beauty is that they capture the essence of the plant in a concentrated form and when turned into a roll-on or spray can be used to heal emotionally.

Always blend "hot" oils with twice as much olive oil or alcohol. Lavender is a calmative and helps skin and sleep, so lavender essential oil will do the same when made into cream. Sandalwood is grounding and is a prayerful herb and is great in a roll-on to apply to pressure points before prayer.

This is a sacred blend of oils to use before meditation, to bless someone before ceremony, or to use before bed to prevent nightmares. It dispels negative energy and the blend of oil balances each chakra.

Sacred Oil Blend

3 drops each:

Lavender

Cedar

Sage

Mint

Rose

Orange

Jasmine

Sandalwood

Add to the blend 2 teaspoons of olive, rose hip, or sunflower oil. Prepare in a ½ dropper bottle, roll-on bottle, or small vessel and apply with finger tips to the top of the head, the forehead, throat, heart, diaphragm (in between and at the base of the lungs), pelvic bone, and tail bone. Putting it on your wrists helps you to smell it during prayers and meditation.

You can also apply this mixture to a child's back before bed and to their heart to prevent night terrors. This blend is especially protective.

The Medicine Person's Guide to Herbalism

9. Healing with Animal Spirits

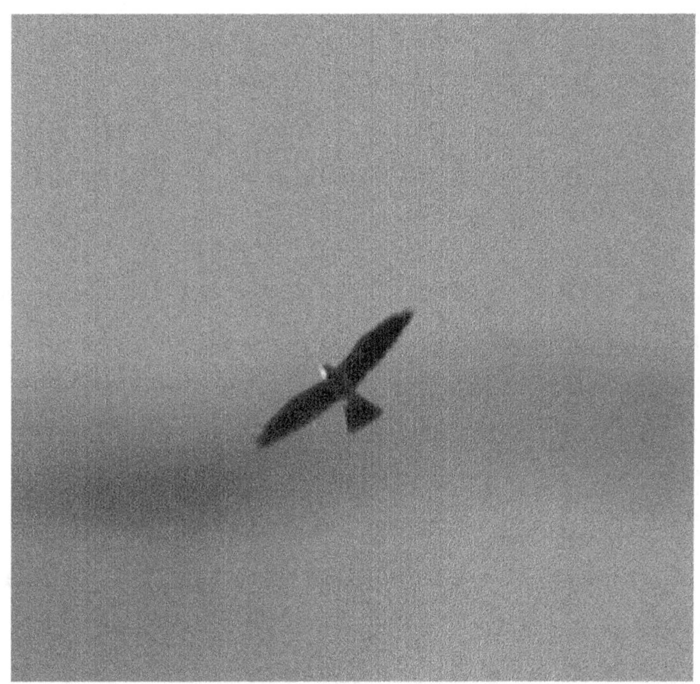

We are just the listeners, the earth keepers, the healers. We have many helpers to assist us on this journey. Animals are one of them. Animals are the very kind, old souls that are far wiser than we are. They will often come to bring us messages to help guide us. Or will offer something of their spirit to help us in ceremony or in medicine. We must always be grateful, mindful, and aware. Offer tobacco or bowls of water or other gifts in return.

You might look around forever and never find a feather when you want one, but then one day you will find several, or maybe just one really special one. Feathers have a way of finding the medicine persons and by looking up what that bird's messages and gifts are, you can utilize it in your work. A Comanche Holy Elder and great friend of mine, who taught me many things about ceremony and healing, taught me that our prayers are lifted on the smoke of our prayers (smudge) and get caught on the feathers of the birds flying overhead and then are taken to the Creator. When a feather drops, it still is sacred and contains the power of the bird and the prayers upon it.

One might find a wing or a part of an animal that stemmed from an unfortunate accident, but those work as well in your work if you ask the animal to help you. I have the wing of a crow and it helps those that are going through a transformation and rebirth of sorts to complete that cycle during ceremony.

Lately, all I have been seeing are Turkey Vultures. They symbolize death/rebirth. I know my work is shifting, changing, just as my life has this last year. One year all I saw were owls and we had the most transformative year of our lives! My friend is being visited by Golden Eagles. It is not a coincidence. One day, a few years ago, my husband and I walked outside our house to find dozens of Bald Eagles flying over our house. Our neighbors could not see them until we pointed them out. They

    The Medicine Person's Guide to Herbalism

were a message for us. If you see a deer or a hummingbird, look up the meaning. Or if one comes to you in a dream, look up the message. Of course, if you live in a neighborhood swarming with deer, then you may wait until you see one alone, or in an unusual place to realize that it is a message for you.

The medicine person will keep a box or bag of sacred objects, many of them having to do with animals, with them during ceremony. The person having the ceremony may be asked to hold a specific feather or the medicine person may don a cloak or headdress with the animal or birds that assist their medicine.

10. Using Stones as Medicine

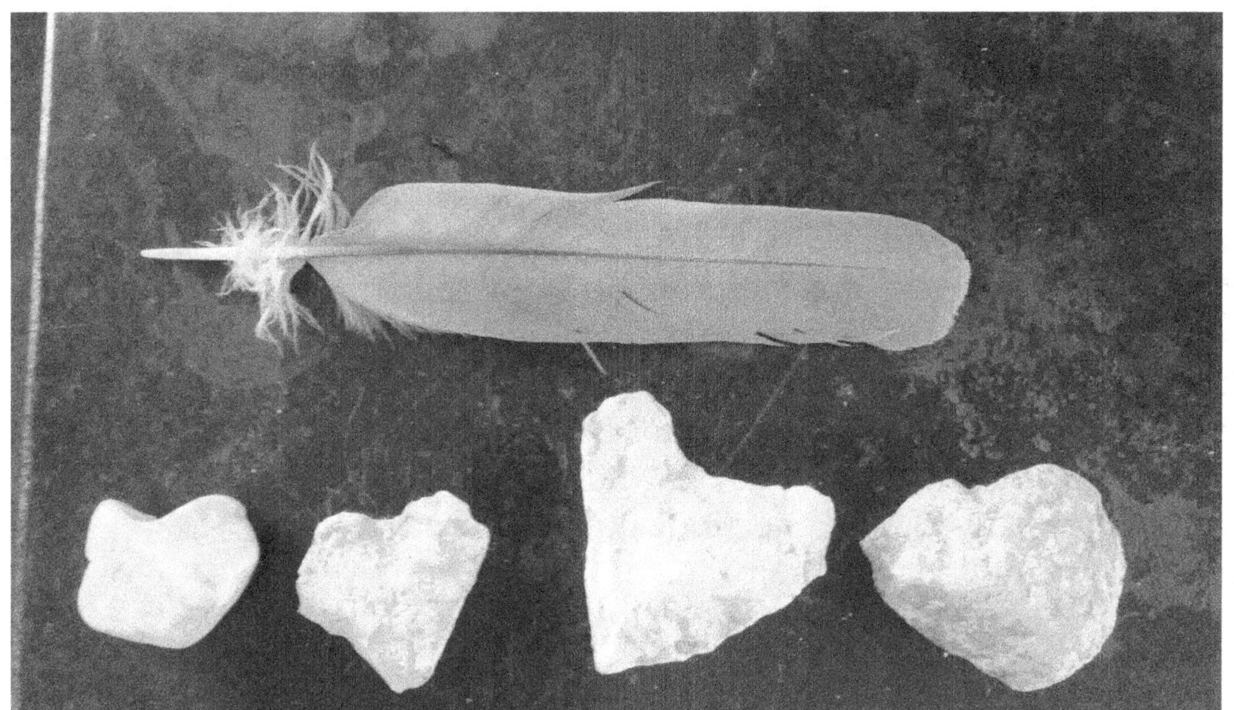

The Rock People are the oldest of the spirits on the earth. My Comanche friend teaches that if it has a shadow, it has a spirit. The Navajo tell tales of rocks rolling thousands of miles to be where they want to be. Indeed, rocks are not inanimate objects, but powerful healers. If asked, they will offer spiritual and physical healing to the seeker.

I performed a healing ceremony for a woman who worked with stones making jewelry and had a great love for them. I did not know this before but felt quite strongly that I needed to use stones during her ceremony. I walked her out and then went back inside. Shortly after, I went outside again and there in the middle of the path was a large stone! I did not put it there and I had a fenced yard, so no one else did either. That was a magical place where I lived, and the stones often moved around untouched and shared their magic.

When I go on walks and feel connected with the nature, I come across sand stones shaped like hearts; like little love notes from the earth.

Just as plants have specific medicinal properties, so do stones. Some heal the heart, some heal blockages in the intestines, and some protect the medicine person from evil spirits.

I was on a meditation journey, through an area in my mind that looks like the forest, and I go through a door and I am in my own sacred place. A place with gnomes and I can shape shift into an owl, and I hear messages. I often wondered if it was just my imagination until one particular event.

The gnomes told me that I needed a healing stone called gypsum. What is gypsum? I wondered. My husband and I were taking a trip to New Mexico that week and we stopped at many places selling rocks. I would ask if they had gypsum and they would reply no. That didn't stop me from picking up certain

                    The Medicine Person's Guide to Herbalism

rocks that appealed to me. It wasn't until we got to the college in Socorro, which has an amazing geology department, that I saw what gypsum was. Its other name is Selenite. As I pulled open my pouch of stones I had collected, I realized that each one was Gypsum!

There are various ways to utilize the medicine of stones. One can brew one into a tea then remove it before drinking. One can place it in medicine that is brewing in the full moon. One can place it in water and brew it outdoors during a full moon (or new moon if it is for a new venture) and drink the water like holy water.

A person having a ceremony can hold the rocks during the healing. One can also carry different stones in a medicine bag or wear them as jewelry.

                                        The Medicine Person's Guide to Herbalism

11. Ceremony for Healing

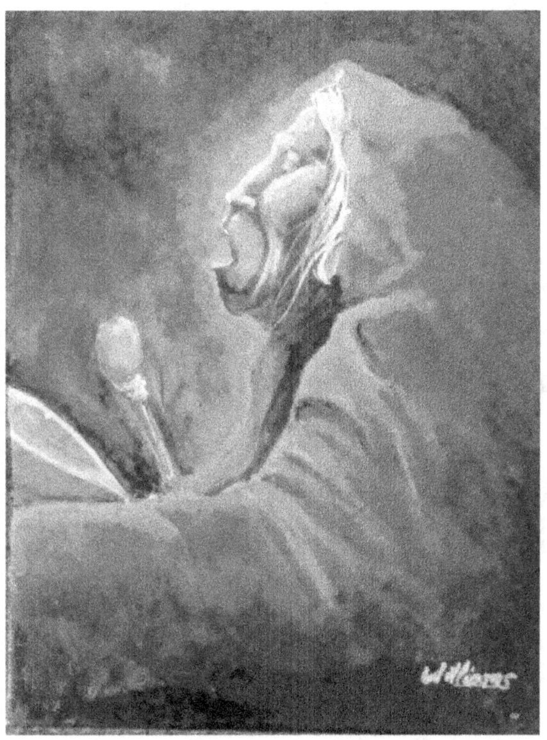

Painted by Thompson Williams, my dear friend and mentor.

Ceremony is a sacrament of sorts. We go through certain motions to increase the power of healing. By using herbs, traditions, prayers, smoke, feathers, animal totems, and other things, like water or a medicine staff, we set the tone for the healing that is to take place. This helps the person receiving ceremony to relax, to accept, and to be healed. For it is their choice whether they will be or not.

Always start with a circle. The circle can be made of tobacco, candles, or stones. This is a place of protection. All of the items needed for the healing are inside of the circle. Sometimes things come to watch, or things are released from the person and they cannot be in the protective circle.

Smudge is a powerful way to pray. There is a common myth that one uses sage to smudge. Even though sage is used, it is never used alone. Just like we don't use single herbs as medicine, we don't use single herbs to pray.

Cedar- cedar is pleasing to the Great Spirit.

Sage- sage (pasture sage, culinary, or ceremonial sage all work) clears negative energy and spirits.

Tobacco- is an offering to the spirits to help us.

Sweet Grass- closes the portals that sage opened and seals everything with positivity and light.

Indian Tobacco- also knowns as Lobelia, this is an herb that can be used with or in place of tobacco. It is a strong prayer herb for serious matters.

Other herbs like rose or lavender or bear root- can be added to specify prayers for love, protection, or physical healing.

   The Medicine Person's Guide to Herbalism

Use a heat proof container, like the Abalone shell (which is shaped like a heart inside), a cast iron pan or small cauldron, or a well fired ceramic bowl. Place your herbs within and use a lighter to set the herbs on fire, releasing the smoke into the atmosphere. If you are performing a longer ceremony, charcoal, specifically for that use, can be placed in the bowl and lit beforehand.

Use a feather that is powerful to you to push the smoke around the space, cleansing the area, the circle, yourself, and the person that is going through ceremony.

A bowl of water with a little tobacco can be placed in the circle to catch negativity. You can even have the recipient of the ceremony wash their face and hands afterwards in fresh water with a pinch of tobacco in it.

Remember, ceremonies change over time depending on place, memory, and custom. You may hear songs, feel like drumming, dance, use bells, or say prayers that come to you. There is no wrong way to do ceremony. There are traditions, but these things evolve with time.

Another way to do ceremony is more private, using candles. There are small, tapered candles that are used for this. I call them witch candles, but you will find them in holistic stores or on line. They come in various colors depending on what you are praying for or what chakra is affected. Use the end of an unbent safety pin to carve in a word or two that denotes your prayer. Light and let burn completely.

Sometimes an outdoor fire with friends can be healing. Choose a night with a full moon or other wonderous astrological event and serve snacks and drinks. Each person can write down what they hope to achieve, what their prayer is, or what they want to release. Each in turn puts their slips of paper in the fire.

    The Medicine Person's Guide to Herbalism

Creating an alter can help you feel connected. Candles, symbols, stones, natural elements, photographs of loved ones and ancestors, incense, and totems are all lovely ways to create ceremony.

However, you choose to do ceremony, wear smoky quartz or other protective stone, smudge yourself off, wear a medicine bag (place in it the sacred herbs and other totems that you identify with like stones or trinkets), and keep a joyous heart. Know that you are not the one healing, but rather the great universe and beyond and the Creator (Goddess, God, Spirit; whatever name you use) is healing through you.

As a medicine person, you must stay true to your sacred path and medicine. You must take great care of yourself. Eat healthy, create a routine and a spiritual practice, cleanse, smudge, learn from other healers, but trust your inner wisdom.

This book will help you along your journey. Learning how plants, trees, stones, animals, and divine guidance work to help you heal others and yourself is a gift, and is a lifetime of learning.

You have the passion, the compassion, the touch, the sight, the hearing, the help of the spirit guides, so let's go. We have healing to do.

About the Author

Katie Lynn Sanders, also known as Bird Woman, is a Cherokee/Celtic Medicine Woman, Master Herbalist, Medical Intuitive, and teacher of herbalism and shamanic practice. She lives with her husband on their homestead, Pumpkin Hollow Farm, in Colorado surrounded by wild plants, mountain views, lots of animals, and their children and grandchildren.

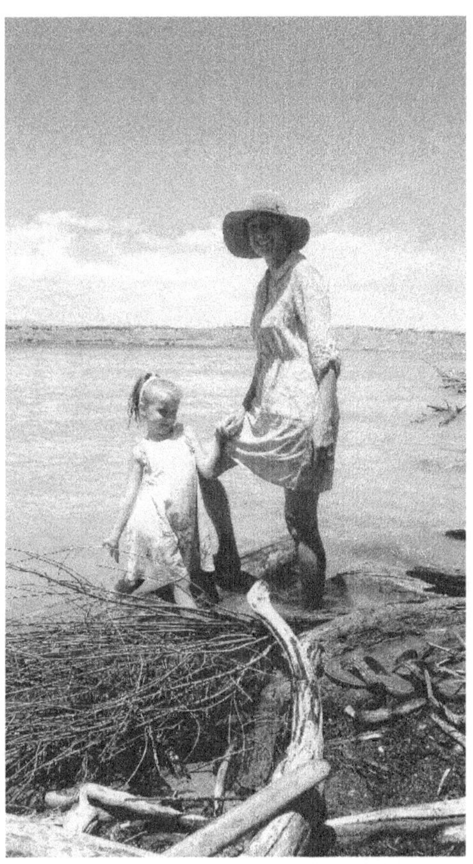

Katie is the founder of White Wolf Medicine and Garden Fairy Apothecary, and author of the popular blog, FarmgirlSchool.org. All of Katie's books can be found at AuthorKatieSanders.com.

www.ingramcontent.com/pod-product-compliance
Lightning Source LLC
Chambersburg PA
CBHW081952260726

48657CB00009BA/2670